The 5:2 Gluten-free Fast Diet

Disclaimer and Terms of Use: Effort has been made to ensure that the information in this book is accurate and complete, however, the author and the publisher do not warrant the accuracy of the information, text and graphics contained within the book due to the rapidly changing nature of science, research, known and unknown facts and internet. The Author and the publisher do not hold any responsibility for errors, omissions or contrary interpretation of the subject matter herein. This book is presented solely for motivational and informational purposes only. Consult your doctor before you engage in any diet or exercise program.

Table of Contents

To say **Thank You** I have prepared some very special FREE gifts for you! They include:

→Printable two week sample menu plans from the book which include breakfast, lunch, dinner, snacks and also a helpful 'do ahead' - a list of prep which will make the next week or day less time consuming!

→10 EXTRA recipes for your non-fasting days, including Homemade Granola Bars, My go to Gluten-free Bread, Baked Cajun Salmon and, Chicken & Broccoli Bake

→10 tips for staying focused on your fast days.

→An extra special treat recipe: Carrot and Pecan Muffins which are both healthy AND tasty!

Grab yours by visiting www.thehealthylifecenter.com and entering your email address and I will send them on to you.

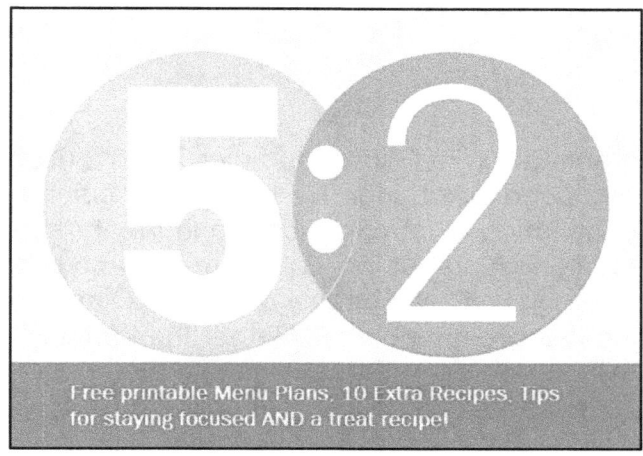

Introduction

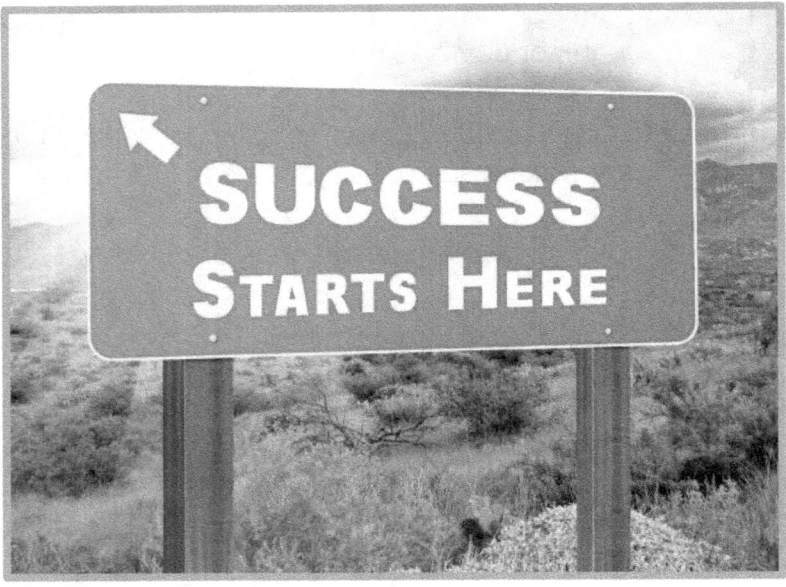

If you are tired of trying and failing to follow a fad diet, the 5:2 Gluten-free Fast Diet may be just the thing you have been looking for. Reducing your calorie intake for a days or weeks on end can be exhausting – both physically and mentally. Eventually you are going to get bored of eating nothing but low-calorie meals and watching your friends indulge in treats you once enjoyed. The beauty of the 5:2 Diet is that you can still enjoy your favorite foods – and lose weight doing it! Rather than forcing yourself through an endless string of days where you eat a reduced calorie diet, the 5:2 Gluten-free Fast Diet encourages you to eat a reduced calorie diet only 2 days a week and to engage in healthy eating habits for the other 5 days. Throughout this book you will learn the basics about the 5:2 Diet as well as the benefits of combining this diet with the vegan diet to achieve your weight loss goals.

There are hundreds, if not thousands, of before and after images on the internet of people who have lost weight on the 5:2 diet. Below is just one of them. It is of Debi and Paul who lost four and a half and one and a half stone respectively on the 5:2 diet. The images are courtesy of The Daily Mail where they were featured.

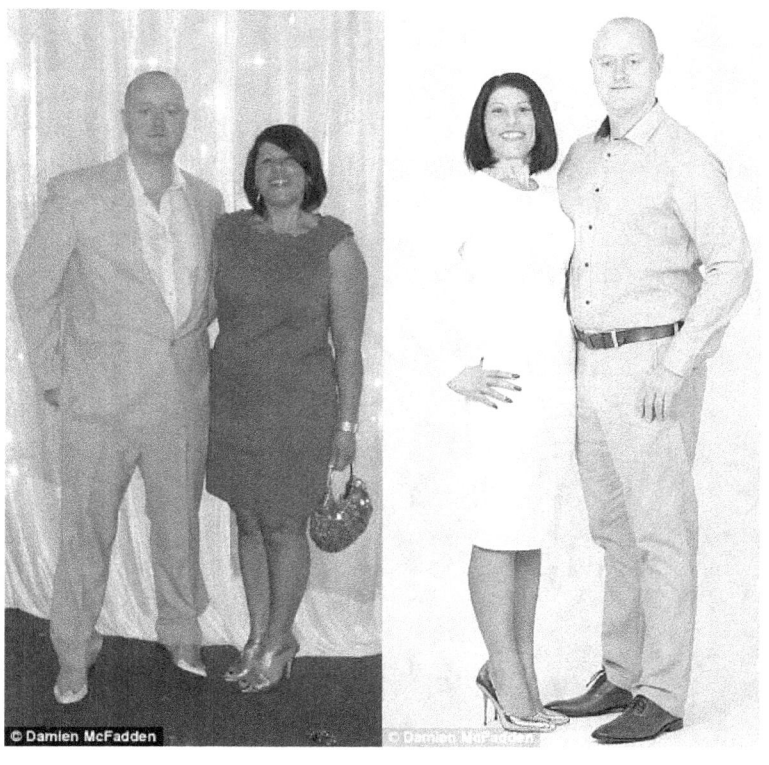

Chapter One: Basics of the 5:2 Diet

"When I first heard about the 5:2 diet I was skeptical. What sparked my interest was the attitude of my friends. This diet is the only one they can bear doing, and what's more, it's working! Science is not conclusively in support of fasting, and neither am I - longer-term fasting can interfere with the immune system and vital bodily functions and can damage the liver, kidneys and other organs. However, the 5:2 diet is not about total fasting – it allows 500 calories a day for women and 600 calories a day for men, two days a week."

- Juliet Gellatley, BSc, Dip CNM, Dip DM, FNTP, NTCC

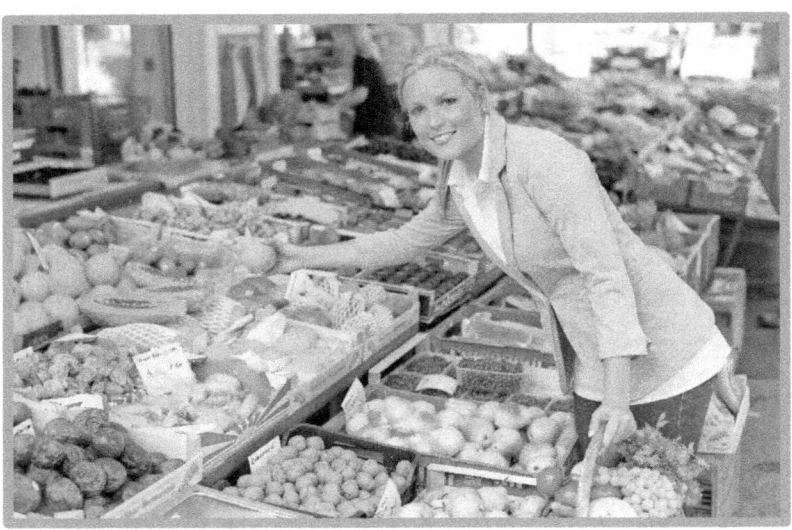

What is the 5:2 Diet?

The 5:2 Diet goes by a number of different names including the Fast Diet – it is also simply referred to as intermittent fasting of IF for short. Do not let the term "fasting" scare you away from this diet because you are not required to fast completely from food at all. The term intermittent fasting simply means that you eat a reduced calorie count on 2 days out of the 7 each week – each week you will have 5 non-fasting days and 2 fasting days. Sounds simple, right? That's because it is. The 5:2 Diet allows you to enjoy your regular eating habits 5 days a week while encouraging a reduced calorie intake on the remaining two non-consecutive days each week.

The practice of fasting has been around since the 1940's but catapulted to 'fame' in the UK when the BBC broadcast an episode on Horizon called 'Eat Fast and Live Longer' in August 2012.

If you are used to following fad diets that prescribe extreme restrictions or specific calorie counts, the 5:2 Diet may seem strange to you. How can you possibly lose weight by only reducing your calorie count twice a week? The 5:2 Diet encourages healthy eating all the time to complement your reduced calorie count twice a week – you will learn more about how intermittent fasting works later in this chapter. For now, however, you may be wondering why the 5:2 Diet is so great. <u>Below you will find a list of the benefits that people following the 5:2 Diet have experienced</u>:

- Healthy weight loss and improved eating habits
- Improved cardiovascular health
- Regulated metabolism – reduced problems with overeating
- Decreased risk for serious diseases (ex: cancer, diabetes, etc.)
- Increased rate of fat loss (especially during fasting periods)
- Reduced inflammation and lowered blood pressure

The Gluten-free 5:2 Diet

The Gluten-free 5:2 Fast Diet is simply a variation of the traditional 5:2 Diet – you still follow the principles of eating normally 5 days a week and fasting twice, but you follow a gluten-free diet all 7 days of the week. The Gluten-free 5:2 Fast Diet is a great alternative to the 5:2 Diet if you have a gluten or wheat intolerance or if you prefer to eat a low carb diet. I myself am gluten-free and when I follow the Gluten-free 5:2 Fast Diet I find you can eat more when not eating gluten or wheat. You get more for your 500 calories for women and 600 calories for men when wheat and some carbs are not involved.

While you already know the basics about the 5:2 Diet, you may not be familiar with the gluten-free diet. In short, this diet eliminates products containing wheat AND gluten. If this sounds a little extreme to you, you will be glad to know that there are plenty of gluten-free friendly food products out there! As an alternative to wheat there are lots of gluten-free flours readily available now in supermarkets like almond flour, oat flour, buckwheat flour, coconut flour and rice flour. The list really is endless. Most supermarkets have a 'Free From' aisle and some even have a 'Free From' freezer section which is great for not just people diagnosed with celiac (coeliac) disease but anyone with a gluten, wheat and dairy intolerance also. Later in this book you will receive a collection of fantastic recipes that will show you just how easy and delicious it can be to follow a gluten-free diet.

If the 5:2 Diet is so effective on its own, you may be wondering why it is necessary to remove gluten also. Studies have shown that following a gluten-free diet can have the following beneficial effects:

1. Improved digestion and digestive function – required for effective weight loss
2. Excess fluid and weight loss
3. Increased energy
4. Better bowel function
5. Improved mental function and better mood
6. Improved sleeping pattern

How Intermittent Fasting Works

You already know that the 5:2 Diet requires you to eat normally 5 days a week and to eat a reduced calorie count on the remaining two days. Given this basic understanding, you are ready to get into the details of the diet. The 5:2 Diet is based on the principle of intermittent fasting – that is, alternating between periods of eating normally and eating a reduced calorie intake. It is recommended that you schedule your fasting days on non-consecutive days each week. For example, you might choose Tuesday and Thursday or Monday and Wednesday – you can choose any two days you like as long as they are not in a row.

When it comes to fasting days, you should aim to consume about 500 calories throughout the course of the day for women and 600 for men. Ideally, you should consume several small meals throughout the day to control your hunger and to keep your metabolism active. For example, you might eat two 200-calorie meals (one in the morning and one in the evening) along with a 100-calorie snack or two 50-calorie snacks spaced throughout the day. It may seem complicated at first, but after a few fasting days you will get the hang of it.

Now that you know how to incorporate intermittent fasting into your diet, you may be curious to know exactly how it works to help you lose weight. Numerous studies have shown that the only way to lose weight is to create a calorie deficit – that is, taking in fewer calories than you expend throughout the course of the day. This deficit can be accomplished by reducing the number of calories you eat or by increasing your calorie expenditure through exercise – or a combination of both. The idea behind intermittent fasting is that reducing your calorie count twice a week will give you a calorie deficit for the week and, hopefully, will encourage you to engage in healthier eating habits even on non-fasting days. When you have the freedom to eat as you choose 5 days a week, you will be less tempted to overindulge.

Chapter Two: 100-Calories or less Dishes

The recipes included in this chapter are all 100 calories or less made up of salads, soups, a smoothie recipe and fruit salad. This makes them a great option for a small meal or a snack during your fasting days. It is important to eat several small meals throughout the day to keep your metabolism going, so keep these delicious recipes on hand! Calories are PER SERVING.

Thai Beef Salad

This is a super tasty and quick salad using beef, chili and lime dressing and at 100 calories it is excellent for fast days!

Servings: 1
Prep: 5 minutes
Cook: 10-15 minutes
Calories: 100

Ingredients:
2 oz lean top sirloin steak - trimmed
¼ red onion – sliced
2 inch cucumber – cut in to matchsticks
½ lemongrass stalk – chopped finely
2 tsp spring onion – chopped
Juice of ½ a lime
½ tbsp fish sauce
1-2 red chilies – finely sliced
Fresh cilantro – to garnish
Cress and Mint leaves to serve

Instructions:

1. Grill or griddle the steak until medium rare – or how you prefer your steak, and allow to rest for 10 minutes. Once cooled cut the steak in to thin slices and put in to a bowl
2. In to the bowl add the cucumber, onions, lemongrass, spring onions and toss with the lime juice and fish sauce.
3. Serve garnished with the cress and mint and garnished with the chili slices and cilantro. This is delicious served chilled or at room temperature.

Crab and Cabbage Salad

So quick and easy to prepare this tasty salad will keep the hunger pangs at bay until your bigger meal of the day.

Servings: 1
Prep Time: 20 minutes
Cook Time: 0
Calories: 98

Ingredients:
¼ cup shredded cabbage
2 tbsps. shredded red cabbage
1/8 head fresh broccoli - broke into florets
1/8 green bell pepper, sliced thinly
1/8 red bell pepper – sliced thinly
½ red onion – sliced thinly
2 ounces crabmeat, coarsely chopped
1 ½ tbsps. light mayonnaise
1 ½ tsps. lemon juice
1 tsp white wine vinegar
1/8 clove garlic - crushed
1/8 tsp Worcestershire sauce
1/8 tsp sea salt
1/8 teaspoon ground black pepper
1/8 teaspoon hot pepper sauce

Instructions:

1. In a small bowl, whisk together mayonnaise, lemon juice, white wine vinegar, garlic, Worcestershire sauce, seasoning, and hot pepper sauce.
2. In a large bowl combine all the veggies and crabmeat. Toss mixture with dressing. Cover, and refrigerate until ready to serve.

'Cream' of Cauliflower Soup

Creamy and thick but so low in calories this soup is hearty and filling while leaving you with enough calories to have larger dish later in the day.

Servings: 4
Prep: 5 minutes
Cook: 0
Calories: 100

Ingredients:
½ tbsp olive oil
1 medium head cauliflower, chopped
1 medium yellow onion, chopped
1 tsp minced garlic
Salt and pepper to taste
4 cups vegetable stock
2 tsps. fresh chopped dill

Instructions:

1. Heat the oil in a large saucepan over medium-high heat.
2. Stir in the onion and cook for 5 minutes.
3. Add the garlic and cook for 1 minute longer.
4. Stir in the remaining ingredients and bring to a boil.
5. Reduce heat and simmer, covered, for 20 minutes until the cauliflower is very tender.
6. Remove from heat and puree the soup in batches in a food processor blender until smooth.
7. Garnish each bowl of soup with ½ teaspoon fresh dill to serve.

Carrot and Cilantro Soup

Soup is great for keeping you full and it is low calorie when the correct ingredients are used. Soup also freezes really well so make a big batch of your favorite type and freeze in to smaller portions.

Servings: 6 – freeze the remainder until your next fast
Prep: 5 minutes
Cook: 20 minutes
Calories: 76.5

Ingredients:
2 tbsp olive oil
1 medium yellow onion – chopped
2 small white potatoes – cut in to small dice
1 celery stick – chopped
1lb carrots – chopped
4 cups chicken stock
2-3 tsp ground cilantro (coriander)
1 tbsp fresh cilantro (coriander)
1 cup semi skimmed milk
Sea salt and freshly ground black pepper

Instructions:

1. Heat the oil in a saucepan over medium heat then add the onion and cook for 3-4 minutes until translucent but not brown.
2. Add the celery, carrots and ground cilantro and cook over a gentle heat for 4 minutes, stirring all the time so nothing sticks to the pan.
3. Add the stock and bring to the boil. Simmer for 5 minutes then add in the diced potato, cook for a further 8-10 minutes or until the potato and carrots are tender.
4. Blend the soup and pour back in to the saucepan. Add the milk, fresh cilantro and taste for seasoning. Garnish with extra cilantro if required.

Roasted Tomato Soup

This is my go to soup not just on fast days but also when it's cold outside and need some comforting. I always make this when I feel a cold or flu coming on also.

Servings: 2
Prep: 5 minutes
Cook: 16 minutes
Calories: 78

Ingredients:
1 tablespoon olive oil
3 medium ripe tomatoes, cored and chopped
1 medium yellow onion, chopped
1 teaspoon minced garlic
2 cups vegetable broth
1 teaspoon dried basil
¼ teaspoon dried oregano
Salt and pepper to taste

Instructions:

1. Heat the oil in a large saucepan over medium-high heat.
2. Add the onion and cook for 5 minutes, stirring occasionally.
3. Stir in the garlic and cook for 1 minute.
4. Add the tomatoes, vegetable broth, basil and oregano.
5. Season with salt and pepper to taste then bring to a boil.
6. Reduce heat and simmer, covered, for 10 minutes.
7. Remove from heat and puree the soup in batches in a food processor or blender.
8. Adjust seasonings as needed and serve hot.

Hot and Sour Prawn Soup

This soup reminds me of when I was in Thailand. The flavors explode in your mouth and will take you back to Phuket (well, for me anyway) If you would like to make this more substantial add some shredded chicken breast.

Servings: 2
Prep: 5 minutes
Cook: 8-10 minutes
Calories: 49

Ingredients:
½ lb King prawns
2 cups chicken stock
1 lemon grass stalk
5 kaffir lime leaves
4oz straw mushrooms (½ 8oz can) See Note
1 ½ tbsp fish sauce
2 tbsp lime juice
1 tbsp spring onions – chopped
½ tbsp fresh coriander – chopped
2 red or green chilies – de-seeded and chopped
Sea salt and freshly ground black pepper

Instructions:

1. Remove the shells and veins from the prawns. Rinse the shells and put in to a large saucepan. Add the stock and bring to the boil.
2. Break the lemongrass stalk and add to the stock with 3 of the kaffir lime leaves. Bring to a simmer and cook for 5 minutes until the lemongrass stalks change color and the stock is lovely and fragrant.
3. Strain the stock to remove the prawn shells, leaves and lemongrass stalks. Reheat over a medium flame, add the mushrooms and prawns. Once the prawns have turned pink add in the remaining ingredients. Check the soup for seasoning before adding. This will taste typically Thai – spicy, sour, salty and hot!

Note: Straw Mushrooms are very popular in Thailand and can be usually found in cans in Asian markets here in the western world. If you cannot find then you can substitute with other mushrooms.

Strawberry Spinach Smoothie

Servings: 1
Prep: 5 minutes
Cook: 0
Calories: 90

Ingredients:
1 cup fresh baby spinach, packed
1 cups water
½ cup frozen sliced strawberries
½ medium frozen banana, peeled and sliced
1 tbsp natural yogurt

Instructions:

1. Combine all of the ingredients in a blender.
2. Blend on high speed for 30 to 60 seconds until smooth and well combined.
3. Pour the smoothie into glasses and serve immediately.

Tropical Fruit Salad

Fresh fruit – there's not much to say here only that it really fills the gap if you cannot wait for your larger meal of the day!

Servings: 1
Prep: 5 minutes
Cook: 0
Calories: 100

Ingredients:
½ ripe kiwi, peeled and sliced
¼ ripe mango, pitted and diced
¼ medium orange, peeled and sectioned
¼ medium ripe banana, peeled and chopped
A drizzle of honey (less than ½ tsp)
Pinch ground cinnamon

Instructions:

1. Combine the fruit in a serving bowl.
2. Toss with cinnamon and honey and mix until well combined.
3. Cover and chill until ready to serve.

Chapter Three: 200-Calorie or less Dishes

The recipes in this chapter are a little more filling than those in the previous chapter which makes them great for an afternoon meal or a hearty snack. Here you will find recipes for herbed quinoa burgers and stuffed tomatoes as well as tasty treats like blueberry lime sherbet. Remember to budget your calories on fasting days to ensure that you don't eat too much at once and go hungry the rest of the day.

Mediterranean Fish

This dish has such great taste and will make a great lunch as it is only 165 calories! You can add some steamed broccoli and carrots to make it a more substantial dinner (remembering to factor them in to your overall calorie count if using)

Servings: 2
Prep: 5 minutes
Cook: 25 – 30 minutes
Calories: 165 per portion

Ingredients:
2 white fish cutlets about 5oz each
1/3 cup fish stock – to poach the fish
1 bay leaf
Strip of lemon peel
Some black peppercorns

Sauce:
½ of a 14oz can crushed tomatoes
1 garlic clove – crushed
½ tbsp capers
6-8 stoned black olives
Sea salt and freshly ground black pepper

Instructions:

1. To make the sauce pour the tomatoes in to a pan with the garlic, capers and olives season to taste with sea salt and black pepper and cook over a low heat for 15-20 minutes, stir every so often so it doesn't stick to the bottom of the pan.
2. Warm an ovenproof dish in the hot oven to place the fish in when cooked. To cook the fish place them in a large frying pan / skillet and pour over the fish stock. Add the peppercorns, lemon rind and bay leaf. Cover with a lid or tin foil and simmer over a low to medium heat for 10 minutes. The fish should flake easily.
3. Remove the fish with a slotted spoon or fish slice in to the heated dish. Strain the fish stock in to the tomato sauce and bring to the boil. Turn the heat down and allow the sauce to reduce and thicken slightly. Ladle the sauce over the fish and sprinkle with freshly chopped parsley or basil.

Turkey & Tomato Hot Pot

Lean turkey mince is a great source of protein and very low in fat. You can change this dish up by using ground chicken. This recipe serves 4 and is freezer friendly. To reheat allow to defrost before reheating in a saucepan over a low – medium heat.

Servings: 4
Prep & chill: 15 minutes
Cook: 30
Calories: 190

Ingredients:
1 garlic clove – crushed
½ tsp caraway seeds
8oz minced turkey
1 egg white
1 ½ cups chicken stock
1 x 14oz can tomatoes
1 tbsp tomato paste
½ cup rice (wholegrain preferably)
Sea salt & freshly ground black pepper
Fresh basil leaves to garnish

Instructions:

1. Place the turkey, garlic, caraway seeds and seasoning to a bowl and mix well.
2. Whisk the egg white in a separate bowl until stiff then fold in to the turkey mixture. Place in the fridge to chill for 10 minutes
3. Meanwhile place the stock, tomatoes and tomato paste in to a saucepan over a medium to high heat.
4. Once the sauce is boiling add the rice, stir and bring back to the boil. Then turn the heat down and allow the sauce to simmer.
5. Remove the turkey mixture from the fridge and shape in to 16 even small balls. Place them carefully in to the sauce and simmer for 8-10 minutes or until the rice is tender and the turkey balls are cooked through.
6. Serve garnished with the fresh basil leaves.

Ragout of Veal

This is a great low calorie dish which is quick to make and perfect for fasting or non-fasting days! If you prefer you can substitute the veal for lean beef or pork fillet.

Servings: 2
Prep: 5 minutes
Cook: 20-25 minutes
Calories: 158

Ingredients:
6oz fillet or loin of veal – fat removed and cut in to cubes
1 tsp olive oil
5-6 shallots
½ each red and orange bell peppers – cut in to large chunks
2 beef tomatoes – peeled and quartered
1 tbsp dry martini (optional)
Handful fresh basil leaves
Sea salt & freshly ground black pepper

Instructions:

1. Heat the oil in a skillet before adding the whole shallots and veal, stir-fry for a couple of minutes.
2. Next add the peppers and tomatoes, stir-fry for a further 5 minutes.
3. Add the martini (if using) season with salt and pepper and add half the basil leaves. Cook on a low heat for 10 – 15 minutes or until the veal is tender.
4. To serve sprinkle over the remaining basil.

Hedgehog Garlic Potato

With this low fat and low calorie topping these baked potatoes, also known as hassle back potatoes, are super tasty. They are great on their own but are also a great accompaniment to meat and fish dishes!

Servings: 1
Prep: 5 minutes
Cook: 1 ¼ hours
Calories: 195 calories

Ingredients:
1 baking potato
1 garlic clove – sliced thinly
2 tbsp low fat natural yogurt
½ tbsp chives - chopped

Instructions:

1. Pre-heat oven to 400F / 200C
2. Slice the potato at ¼ inch intervals about ¾ the way down the potato (we want them to keep their shape while cooking)
3. Add the garlic slices to the cuts in the potato and place on a roasting tin. Bake for 1 – 1 ¼ hours or until the potato is cooked.
4. To make the topping add the yogurt to a bowl with the chives and add some black pepper to taste.
5. Place a dollop of the yogurt on top of the potato and devour!

Chicken Curry

Who doesn't love a nice curry and at 152 calories per portion (without sides) this is a perfect fast day dish. Lentils are an excellent source of fiber too! This makes 4 servings and you can be easily froze for next week's fast days.

Servings: 4
Prep: 5 minutes
Cook: 35 minutes
Calories: 152

Ingredients:
2 chicken breasts, skin removed and cut in to large cubes
½ cup red lentils
2 tbsp milk curry powder
2 tsp ground cilantro
1 tsp cumin seeds
1 tbsp fresh cilantro plus extra to garnish
8oz fresh spinach - chopped
Sea salt & freshly ground black pepper

Instructions:

1. Place the lentils in a sieve and rinse under cold running water before putting in to a large sauce pan with the cumin, coriander, curry powder and stock. Bring to the boil before lowering the heat, cover and simmer for 10 minutes.
2. Next add in the chicken and cover. Cook on a low heat for 20 minutes before adding the spinach then cook for a further 5 minutes until the spinach has wilted.
3. Add the fresh cilantro and taste for seasoning, serve with extra cilantro sprinkled on top. If you have spare calories or are having this on a non-fasting day serve with poppadum's (ensure they are traditional ones made with lentil flour) and some wholegrain rice.

Chili Chicken Burger

You can get ground chicken easily in most supermarkets nowadays. However, you can make your own by whizzing chicken breasts in a food processor. These also taste great cooked on a barbeque.

Servings: 2
Prep: 10 minutes
Cook: 10
Calories: 149

Ingredients:
½ lb ground chicken
1 clove garlic – crushed
½ red chili – chopped finely
½ tbsp fresh mint leaves – chopped
1 tbsp fresh parsley – chopped
1 tsp Worcestershire sauce (ensure it is GF)
Olive oil for brushing the burgers
Sea salt and freshly ground black pepper

Instructions:

1. Pre-heat your broiler to medium.
2. In a bowl mix the chicken, garlic, chili, herbs, Worcestershire sauce, sea salt and freshly ground black pepper.
3. With damp hands shape the mixture in to two burgers and brush lightly with oil.
4. Broil for 5 minutes on each side until cooked through and golden in color.

Charred Peaches and Feta Salad

This is what I call a 'taste sensation salad'. I eat this all the time, on fast and non-fast days! This serves 4 as anyone that sees you making this will want it too, I guarantee. It's easily adjusted if you are making it for one.

Servings: 4
Prep: 10 minutes
Cook: 3 minutes
Calories: 198

Ingredients:
1 tsp olive oil
3 ripe peaches – de-stoned and cut in to wedges
Zest and juice of 1 lime
7oz bag of mixed salad leaves
1 red onion – sliced thinly
5oz sugar snap peas – cut in half lengthways
2 tbsp freshly chopped mint
7oz feta cheese – crumbled gently with your hands
Freshly ground black pepper

Instructions:
1. Place the peach wedges in to a bowl and pour over the lime juice. Heat half the oil in a frying pan or brush on to a griddle pan.
2. When the pan starts to smoke place the peaches in, cook until they are charred - this will take around 3 minutes.
3. In a large mixing bowl add the salad leaves, onion, sugar snap peas, lime zest, remaining oil, lime juice and mint. Toss to coat everything then divide between 4 serving bowls.
4. Add the charred peaches and crumble over the feta cheese, season with black pepper, serve immediately.

Tarragon Chicken

Creamy and tasty but only 152 calories! Need I say more?!

Servings: 1
Prep: 10 minutes
Cook: 20
Calories: 152

Ingredients:
1 small skinless chicken breast
2 tbsp low-fat natural yogurt
½ tsp wholegrain mustard
1 small garlic clove - crushed
Fresh tarragon leaves
Zest and juice ½ orange
2oz green beans - trimmed
½ fennel bulb - trimmed and sliced

Instructions:

1. Make a few slashes in the chicken with a sharp knife and season with freshly ground black pepper.
2. Place the yogurt, mustard, garlic, tarragon and juice of ¼ orange along with the zest in to a shallow ovenproof dish. Mix together well to combine.
3. Place the chicken in to the marinade and massage to ensure it is all covered.
4. Allow to marinade for 20 minutes at least (overnight if possible).
5. Pre-heat oven to 400F / 200C.
6. Bake the chicken breast in the oven for 20 minutes or until cooked through.
7. Place the green beans and fennel into a microwaveable bowl. Add the remaining juice of the orange and one teaspoon of water.
8. Microwave for 3 minutes then drain and serve with the yummy tarragon chicken.

Chapter Four: 300-Calorie or less Dishes

The recipes in this chapter are a little heartier, designed for your main meal on fasting days. Here you will enjoy dishes like Piri-Piri Pork and Spaghetti Bolognese as well as chili beef tacos. Remember, you should only consume one 300-calorie meal per day so you have enough calories left to split between smaller meals.

Grilled Cajun Steak

Sirloin steak is a very lean meat, however there is a layer of fat around the top edge of each steak which you can trim off before cooking. This dish is quick and very tasty AND only 291 calories.

Servings: 1
Prep: 15 minutes + standing time
Cook: 15 minutes
Calories: 291

Ingredients:
1 x 5oz lean sirloin steak
1 garlic clove
¼ tsp black peppercorns
¼ tsp cumin seeds
½ tsp dried oregano
¼ tsp cayenne pepper
¼ tsp sea salt (coarse)
Zest of half a lemon

For the tomato salad
2 medium plum tomatoes
Handful of fresh mint
Handful of fresh cilantro
½ red onion – sliced thinly
½ green chili – finely chopped
1 tsp olive oil
Juice of ¼ of a lemon
Sea salt & freshly ground black pepper
Leafy greens to serve

Instructions:

1. Using a coffee grinder or pestle and mortar grind up the lemon zest, clove of garlic, black peppercorns and cumin seeds until well combined. Add in the salt, cayenne and dried oregano and whizz or grind again.
2. Spread this mixture all over the steak and rub in well. Allow to marinade for 1-2 hours if possible.
3. Halve the tomatoes and place cut side down in to a hot skillet or griddle pan and allow to cook for 6-8 minutes until they are charred and soft.
4. In a bowl mix the onion, chili, oil, lemon juice and tomatoes. Season to taste before chopping all the fresh herbs and adding to the mixture.

5. Char-grill your steak on a hot griddle pan for 3-4 minutes each side (or longer if you prefer it well done) Serve with the tomato salad and some leafy greens.

Piri-Piri Pork

Piri piri, also known as peri peri and pili pili is most often served with chicken and originates from Portugal. It is also popular in parts of Africa and Brazil. It is spicy and fiery, and packs a real punch. You can of course use store bought sauce of you prefer but homemade is, as always, much better!

Servings: 2
Prep: 15 minutes
Cook: 16 - 20
Calories: 237

Ingredients:

Piri Piri Sauce
10-12 medium size birds eye chilies
1 tsp sea salt flakes
Juice of 1/2 a lemon
3 ½fl oz olive oil
2 tbsp garlic powder
½ tsp paprika
½ tsp oregano

½ lb pork fillet
1 lemon
Oil – for brushing
3 tbsp piri piri sauce
Cocktail sticks (soaked for 20 minutes in water before cooking)

Instructions:

1. To make the Piri-Piri sauce: Preheat oven to 350F and place chilies on to a baking tray and roast for 10 minutes. Once cooled chop roughly and place in to a saucepan with the remaining ingredients, simmer for 3 minutes. Once the mixture has cooled blend in a food processor until smooth. Store in a jar at room temperature. Always shake the mixture before using.
2. Soak 8-10 cocktail sticks in water for 20 minutes.
3. Cut the pork fillet in to rounds half an inch thick and brush with the Piri-Piri sauce. Slice the lemon thinly and brush lightly with some oil. Put a lemon slice on top of each slice of pork and stick in place with a cocktail stick.
4. Cook on a BBQ or hot griddle pan lemon side down first for 3 minutes then turn over and cook for a further 3 minutes.

5. To serve drizzle over some more sauce. You could add some stir fried vegetable to this dish, just remember to add them to your calories for the day if using on a fast day.

Chili Beef Tacos

Chili beef tacos on fast days? Yes it is possible as these come in at just 264 calories per serving. This recipe serves 6 and is a great dish to have in the freezer for the fast days you don't want to cook. This is perfect for non-fast days too, add to a baked potato and top with some grated cheese.

Servings: 6
Prep: 10 minutes
Cook: 30
Calories: 264

Ingredients:
1 tsp vegetable oil
1 yellow onion – finely diced
2 cloves garlic – crushed
2 red chilies – seeded and roughly chopped (leave the seeds in if you like it hotter!)
1lb 2oz lean steak mince (or lean beef mince)
½ tsp cumin seeds
1 tsp Chinese five spice powder
1 tsp paprika
14 oz can chopped tomatoes
1 tbsp tomato paste
14oz can kidney beans – drained
Sea salt & freshly ground black pepper

To serve:
6 corn taco shells
Shredded lettuce
Paprika

Instructions:

1. Dry fry the cumin seeds in a pan until aromatic, then grind to a powder using a pestle and mortar or coffee grinder.
2. Heat the olive oil in a large saucepan before adding the garlic, onion and chilies. Cook for 5 minutes, stirring all the time as to not let the garlic burn as it will go bitter. Add the mince, all the spices and cook for 5 minutes until the mince starts to brown.
3. Next add in the chopped tomatoes, tomato paste and kidney beans, bring the mixture up to the boil then allow to simmer over a low-medium heat for 20-30 minutes. We want a thick and dark chili. Check for seasoning.
4. Take the taco shells and fill with lettuce before topping with the chili, sprinkle over some extra paprika and serve!

Sweet and Sour Fish

Servings: 2
Prep: 5 minutes
Cook: 30
Calories: 255

Ingredients:

2 tbsp cider vinegar
1 ½ tbsp light soy sauce
1/8 cup granulated sugar
½ tbsp tomato paste
1 tbsp corn flour
½ cup warm water
½ green bell pepper – sliced
½ 8oz can pineapple pieces in juice
4oz tomatoes – chopped roughly
1 cup button mushrooms
¾ lb haddock fillets
Sea salt & freshly ground black pepper

Instructions:

1. Preheat oven to 350F / 180C.
2. In a saucepan mix the first four ingredients. Place the corn flour in to a jug then stir in the warm water before adding to the saucepan. Turn the heat to high and bring to the boil, stirring until thickened. Turn the heat down and simmer for 5 minutes
3. Add the pineapple and juices, green peppers, mushrooms and tomatoes to the pan and heat. Season to taste.
4. Place the fish fillets in the bottom of an ovenproof dish then spoon over the sauce. Cover with lid or foil and bake for 15-20 minutes (depending on the thickness of the fish) and serve immediately once cooked.

'Spaghetti' Bolognese

The sauce for this is very similar to our chili beef tacos but without the spice. We will be using fresh and dried herbs for flavor and the spaghetti is zucchini noodles make with a spiralizer or a julienne peeler. Believe me when I say you will love that this serves 6 and you can freeze for the days you don't feel like or have the time to cook!

Servings: 6
Prep: 5 minutes
Cook: 50 minutes
Calories: 300

Ingredients:
1 tsp vegetable oil
1 yellow onion – finely diced
1 large carrot – peeled and diced
2 cloves garlic – crushed
1lb 2oz lean steak mince (or lean beef mince)
½ tsp cumin seeds
1 tsp dried oregano
1 tbsp fresh parsley
1 tsp paprika
14 oz can chopped tomatoes
1 tbsp tomato paste
2 cups beef stock
Sea salt & freshly ground black pepper
2 medium zucchini – made in to noodles

Instructions:
1. Heat the oil in a large skillet over low-medium heat.
2. Stir in the onion and carrot and cook for 4-5 minutes.
3. Add the garlic and cumin seeds and cook for 2-3 minutes, making sure not to burn the garlic.
4. Add the lean steak mince, breaking up as you cook it so there are no large lumps.
5. Next add the tomato paste, tinned tomatoes, beef stock, paprika and oregano.
6. Bring to the boil before reducing the heat and allow to simmer for 35 to 40 minutes until the sauce has thickened. Taste for seasoning
7. Steam or stir-fry the zucchini 'spaghetti' before placing in to a bowl and topping with Bolognese.

Fishcakes with Chili Lemon Mayo

Easy to prepare and filling! These are great for non-fasting days also. Just add some homemade sweet potato oven baked fries and a tossed salad.

Servings: 2
Prep: 5 minutes
Cook: 10
Calories: 300

Ingredients:
½ celery stick - diced
1 spring onion (scallion) - chopped
2 tbsp fresh parsley leaves
8oz white fish fillets, (such as halibut / hake) roughly chopped
1 organic rice cake - whizzed up to a powder (this acts as our breadcrumbs)
1/2 egg
1 tsp Dijon mustard
1/8 tsp pepper
1 tbsp vegetable oil

Chili Lemon Mayo
2 tbsp light mayonnaise
1 tbsp lemon juice
Pinch chili powder

Instructions:

1. Put the celery, green onions and parsley in to a food processor and whizz until finely chopped.
2. Scrape into bowl with a spatula. Next, place the fish into food processor and whizz until fine. Add to bowl then mix in rice cake crumbs, egg, mustard and pepper.
3. Shape in to 4 even patties about 1/2 inch thick.
4. Heat the oil in a non-stick pan and add the fish cakes.
5. Cook for 4-5 minutes each side until firm and golden.
6. To make the lemon chili mayo mix all the ingredients in a bowl until combined and serve with the fishcakes and some tossed greens.

Southwest BBQ Chicken Quesadillas

Quesadillas are easy to prepare and the great thing is you can mix up the vegetables to whatever you have in your fridge.

Servings: 1
Prep: 5 minutes
Cook: 20 minutes
Calories: 280

Ingredients:
1 egg wrap (see instructions)
½ cooked chicken breast - shredded
1 tsp olive oil
½ thinly sliced yellow onion
¼ cup diced red bell pepper
2 tbsp barbecue sauce
¼ tsp chili powder

Instructions:

1. The egg wrap is so simple to make and is a great low calorie, low carb gluten-free alternative. Beat one egg in a bowl and add seasoning. Heat a non-stick skillet over a medium high heat then add the egg, swirling around until the bottoms is covered. Cook for 1-2 minutes before turning over and cooking for a further minute. Voila an egg wrap! Leave to one side while you prepare the filling (these can also be made ahead and kept in the fridge)
2. Heat the oil in a skillet over medium-high heat.
3. Stir in the onions and cook for 5 minutes until they start to brown.
4. Add red bell pepper.
5. Stir in the chili powder and shredded chicken, and cook for another 5 minutes until the vegetables are tender.
6. Meanwhile, spread the barbecue sauce over half the egg wrap.
7. Spoon the chicken and vegetable mixture over the barbecue sauce and fold the other half of the wrap over top.
8. Spray one side of the wrap with cooking spray and add to the hot skillet.
9. Cook for 1 to 2 minutes until browned then repeat with the other side of the quesadilla.
10. Transfer to a plate and cut in to three triangles and serve immediately.

Chapter Five: Sample Meal Plans

Starting a new diet can be very challenging, especially if it involves making some significant changes to your eating habits. Earlier in this book you received a collection of 100-, 200- and 300-calorie dishes to use in getting started on the Vegan 5:2 diet – in this chapter you will receive some sample meal plans incorporating those recipes. For many people, the biggest challenge in sticking to a diet is getting bored with the food. Using the sample meal plans in this section you will find it easy to stick to the Vegan 5:2 diet because you never have to wonder what you will be eating – you will have a set plan for your weekly diet so you know what tasty meals you have to look forward to!

Sample Meal Plan 1

This meal plan uses only recipes from the book for meals on fasting days. For non-fasting days you will find a combination of recipes from the book as well as healthy meals like grilled chicken and vegetable skewers and Lean Moussaka. Recipes not in this book are included in your free gift along with printable versions of the two week meal plans. Feel free to substitute other meals for those listed on the meal plan for non-fasting days according to your preference. Snacks are optional and just there for a guide on non-fasting days.

5:2 Sample Meal Plan Week 1 (FD = Fast Day)

Meals	Monday	Tuesday (FD)	Wednesday	Thursday (FD)	Friday	Saturday	Sunday
Breakfast	Gluten-free Oats (porridge) with seeds	Hot Water and Lemon	Scrambled Eggs, Grilled Bacon & Tomato	Hot Water and Lemon	Mixed Berry Smoothie	Grilled bacon with poached eggs	Gluten-free Oats with mixed berries
Lunch	Tuna Salad with Avocado and Grapes	Strawberry Spinach Smoothie	Homemade Vegetable Soup	Roasted Tomato Soup	Ham, Onion & Cheese Omelete	Chicken caesar salad with GF croutons	Tossed Tuna Salad with Avocado
Dinner	Chili Beef Tacos with Homemade Sweet Potato Oven Fries	Grilled Cajun Steak	Grilled Chicken & Vegetable Skewers served with Quinoa salad	Chili Chicken Burger	Chicken & Broccoli Stir-fry with rice noodles	Moussaka made with lean steak mince	Ragout of Veal with Mashed Potato
Snacks	Yogurt with Kiwi fruit	Tropical Fruit Salad	Granola Bar or an apple	Small Banana	Homemade Granola Bar	Glass of White Wine	
Do Ahead	Monday	Tuesday	Wednesday	Thursday	Friday	Saturday	Sunday
Prep for tomorrow	Make Granola bars for the week.	Make soup and marinade chicken in yogurt and Cajun spices for dinner.	Prepare chicken burgers for tomorrow.				Make Granola bars and a loaf of gluten-free bread for next week.

Sample Meal Plan 2

This meal plan uses only recipes from the book for meals on fasting days. For non-fasting days you will find a combination of recipes from the book as well as healthy meals Chicken & Broccoli Bake and Baked Cajun Salmon which again are included in your free gift along with printable versions of the two week meal plans.

5:2 Sample Meal Plan Week 2 (FD = Fast Day)

Meals	Monday	Tuesday	Wednesday (FD)	Thursday	Friday (FD)	Saturday	Sunday
Breakfast	Grilled bacon on GF Toast	Green Smoothie	Hot water and lemon	Sliced banana on GF Toast	Hot water and Lemon	Grilled bacon with poached eggs	Oatmeal with Maple Syrup
Lunch	Spanish Frittata with Tossed Salad	Butternut Squash & Sweet Potato Soup	Thai Beef Salad	Charred Peaches and Feta Salad	Cream of Cauliflower Soup	Crab and Cabbage Salad	Hedgehog Garlic Potato
Dinner	Baked Cajun Salmon with oven roast Vegetables	Chicken & Broccoli Bake (no cream!)	Chicken Curry	Baked Cod with Homemade Oven Chips & Peas	Mediterranean Fish	Turkey & Tomato Hotpot with extra Vegetables	Tarragon Chicken with Wholegrain Rice or Mashed potatoes and green beans
Snacks	Granola Bar	Granola Bar	Fruit Salad	Small Banana	Strawberry Spinach Smoothie	Hummus and Vegetable sticks	Treat: Carrot & pecan muffins.
Do Ahead	Monday	Tuesday	Wednesday	Thursday	Friday	Saturday	Sunday
Prep for tomorrow (optional)	Prepare Butternut & Sweet potato Soup	Marinade the beef for the salad					Make Granola bars for next week. Make a batch of Soup.

Conclusion

In reading this book, hopefully you have found the answers to your questions about the 5:2 Gluten-free diet. In addition to receiving a basic overview of the diet and its benefits, you received valuable tips for getting started on the diet as well as a collection of up to 100, 200 and 300-calorie recipes to use on your fast days. As an added bonus, you also received two sample weekly meal plans incorporating the recipes included in this book along with a free gift which you can download HERE. Your free gift includes printable versions of the two-week sample meal plans above, recipes for non-fasting days and some more tips for staying on track on fasting days. With this book as your guide you are ready to get started on the 5:2 diet, lose weight and feel healthier. Best of luck!

What are you waiting for? Get started today to see what benefits the 5:2 diet has in store for you!

If you enjoyed this book and have friends or family that are vegan and are interested in the 5:2 diet, I also have a 5:2 Vegan book published.

Sophie Miller

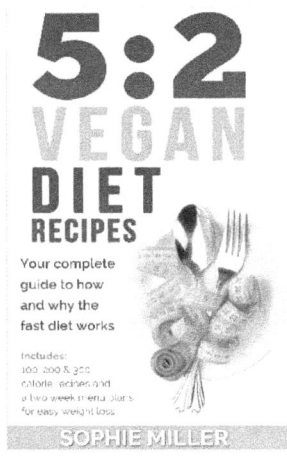